Surviving Cancer:
Lessons to help you win your battle

Clint Seward,
a five year cancer survivor

ISBN 978-0-557-14770-0

Seward Publishing, Inc.
42 Washington Drive
Acton, MA 01720
978 263 3871
cseward@verizon.net

With thanks to

My wife Mary Anne who was with me every day
My neighbor Charlene who saved my life

Table of Contents

Prologue

The tears have finally stopped so I can now tell this story of cancer and paralysis of my legs. For three years, tears would fill my eyes each time I tried to write it. Tears of relief; tears of joy; and tears of thankfulness for all of the great people who helped me in my recovery.

Those three years included three new grandchildren to add to the first three, all living nearby and growing up to be beautiful little kids. It included me learning how to walk again after my doctors were afraid I would not be able to.

My cancer came on so slowly that we all had trouble recognizing it, and my primary care doctor missed it altogether. It started out as a pain in my back, which could have been from heavy chores or just my 60 years of living. But it got worse over the course of a year until I could not walk due to the pain. Things finally got so bad that my neighbor, a nurse, insisted I get to a hospital in spite of what my doctors were telling me. Once there I found the great staff and care that diagnosed me correctly and saved my life. This book recounts that story.

My cancer survival taught me great lessons about cancer, hospitals, rehab, and about myself. I got through it by listening to and following some great advice. Hopefully the lessons I learned can help someone else.

I am convinced I have had a happy ending to my difficulties due mainly to the love and care of my wife and guardian angel Mary Anne.

For every hour I spent in rehab she spent an hour fighting doctors, insurance, government, and everyone else who presented a hurdle to our recovery.

Also, I will always be thankful to my neighbor Charlene who recognized the danger long before any doctors did. Her growing concern and eventual alarm started the process of treatment and recovery within hours of it being too late.

I wish any readers all the best of luck in finding the staff, treatments, and comfort needed to help you with your struggle to survive cancer.

Clint Seward, a cancer survivor.

Chapter 1

A Desperate Situation

The pain kept getting worse for months, but still the cancer caught us by surprise. How did I go from full health, walking 3 miles a day, and jogging several times a week, to paralysis of my legs and near death without anybody noticing? It is not like I had not asked many doctors about the pain in my back and the gradual loss of mobility. Why did it take from February until mid-July for us to get the help we needed? What should we have done differently?

I first noticed continual pain in my back in January. It came after I had shoveled snow and so I naturally assumed a cause and effect. But it persisted and got worse in spite of rest and care. My daughter Ruth arranged a massage session, and the masseuse said right away that the back pain was not normal and that I should see a doctor. I listened, and started my many trips to many doctors, all of whom missed what was happening.

In February I went to my primary care doctor, who quickly concluded I had probably just pulled a muscle and that pain killers should be all I would need. I should see improvement shortly. He also said that it might just be an age related condition since I was over 60, some arthritis of the spine. He sent me to a physical therapy group for treatments twice a week. While this seemed reasonable, it did not help.

After three treatments, one therapist tried to "fix" the "misplaced vertebrate" that she "knew" was the problem. Her aggressive treatments greatly increased the pain because what she targeted was not the problem. Neither she nor my doctor recognized that there was a more serious problem.

I changed physical therapy groups. My new therapist gave me different exercises and they seemed to help. Looking back, the pain in my back would be very bad for a few days, then with pain killers and treatments it would get markedly better. But then about a week later it would get worse again. These cycles of pain then relief then pain would give a temporary sense that things were probably going to get better, but in reality they were getting worse, much, much worse, but too slowly for us to know for sure.

Through March, my doctor still continued the pain killers, but nothing more. He did take an x-ray in his office, but they showed nothing. My surgeon later looked at the x-ray, after the operation, and told me that any reasonable reading of the x-ray would not raise any alarm and would not lead to further actions since the cancer did not show up.

Meanwhile, my neighbor Charlene, a visiting nurse for an insurance company, urged me to get other opinions. Charlene recommended I go to see a chiropractor which I did. She knew many doctors and chiropractors due to her work as a visiting nurse. She recommended a great chiropractor who had helped a lot of her patients to relieve their pain. But after three sessions he said he did not want to do any more work because he could see that the problem was much more serious and that I needed a doctor.

In April my primary care doctor continued the pain killers. He continued to think this was likely an age related issue, either the arthritis that showed on the x-rays, or a slight disc problem that might improve with therapy.

I was able to schedule a session with a major Boston back and spine specialist group, but that led nowhere. They could see no problem. Much later I was able to remember that they had asked, among many questions, if I had any numbness, and although I had a small area of partial numbness on one thigh, I did not understand the importance of what he was asking. So we missed a chance to discover the cancer early on.

The month of May brought more of the same. By now I could not lie down due to the pain in my back. I could only sleep sitting at a table with my head propped up on pillows. Still, my doctor continued to prescribe pain killers and assure me that it would get better. At the end of May the pain was much worse and I had begun to cough incessantly. I visited my doctor's medical group since he was not available that day and the doctor who looked at me at that time prescribed more pain killers, but did not have time to look further. I would need another appointment.

I cannot describe the toll on Mary Anne that this situation was creating. I could not walk very well any more due to the pain, so she would help me onto one of our office chairs with wheels, and then she would push me to get around the house. This loss of mobility created an enormous strain for her to take care of me.

On June 6th, my birthday, all my kids and grand kids came to visit. For the first time in my life I could not get out of my chair to play with my grandkids. My kids and wife were all increasingly alarmed by this, but I was seeing doctors. What more could I do? We all decided we had to figure this out.

In mid June I visited my primary care doctor again. This time I had to use an office wheel chair to get to his office. This did not raise any red flags in his mind. His nurse even dismissed this new turn of events, telling Mary Anne that "men are just babies." The doctor prescribed pain killers and more therapy with a new physical therapy group.

The pain at this point would often shoot through my back and legs and cause me to scream. My new therapist witnessed one of my pain spasms and she immediately called my doctor and told him that on a scale of one to ten my pain was a twenty. I visited my doctor again, but, after an office x-ray, he decided that more pain killers would be sufficient. The pain was so great at this point and the lack of mobility so complete that I could no longer continue with therapy.

Here I got lucky. Charlene, my visiting nurse neighbor, made it a point to stop in every day or so to see how I was doing. She was growing more and more concerned and made sure over the months that I had gone to several different doctors. But this latest bout of pain and immobility raised red flags in her mind, while we continued to trust our doctors. She tried to be very insistent about what needed to be done, without getting us too upset. Her recommendation was to get a visiting nurse in right away to evaluate me. This was a new suggestion my primary care doctor never thought about doing. Mary Anne called his office immediately to get a prescription written.

It was late Friday when she called. The nurse was not happy to receive a request in late afternoon and made that clear. It would take a prescription from a doctor to get a visiting nurse to see us, and the nurse did not think it could be done Friday afternoon. Our primary care doctor took Friday afternoons off and she could not be sure who else could write such a prescription. It turned out the prescription did not get written.

That Saturday my daughters came over to visit and I was not able to get out of my office chair. My wife needed to assist me in the bathroom. My ankles had swelled to 3 times their size, and my thighs were now like jelly. Ruth and Jean then decided that they needed to be there more often to help out and figure out what was going on.

The following Tuesday Charlene stayed home from work and came over to find out what had happened. Jean had come by also since she knew things were getting desperate. Mary Anne said she had just checked with our primary care doctor and the prescription had not been sent in yet. Charlene became insistent. Normally a mild mannered friend, she insisted Mary Anne get on the telephone immediately and stay on it until the visiting nurse came. Do not take "no" for an answer.

I think that was the tipping point when we began to realize how dangerous my situation had become. Mary Anne is very good at getting action through phone calls. She called our doctor's office and got the prescription called in. She then called the visiting nurse facility at Emerson Hospital, a very professional group. When they heard what the situation was, they immediately sent their best visiting nurse over to assess my case.

After fifteen minutes, the visiting nurse looked me straight in the eye and said, "Mr. Seward, you are in a desperate situation. You need a lot of help and you need it right away." I asked how I could get any help when I could not even stand up, let alone get into my car. She said that was easy, picked up the phone and called 911.

In a few minutes the ambulance was there and two large firemen in boots and firefighting gear carried me out to the ambulance. I was on my way to the Emerson Hospital emergency room. This was to be the beginning of a long, long road of treatment and therapy.

But finally, I was in the hands of a medical group and they knew something was terribly wrong. It was not yet clear what or why, but they knew they had to find out quickly. They took x-rays and all the tests they could do, but could not determine a cause. They called in a neurologist, and in a few minutes he determined I had some loss of feeling in a few spots in my thigh. This is a sign of the greatest of serious conditions since it involved nerve damage. They knew we needed an MRI.

But I could not have an MRI since I had not been able to lie down for nearly three months due to the great pain. They needed to find a hospital with an emergency room where I could be anesthetized and then get the MRI. There were only two in Massachusetts: Mass General in Boston and UMASS in Worcester. By now it was getting late, well into the evening, but the staff at Emerson stayed well after their shift ended, knowing how serious this case had become.

Emerson called both hospitals. They each sent an ambulance. Mary Anne said they should leave it in the hands of God as to which hospital we would go to, getting into the first ambulance that came. I am sure we would have done well in either hospital. But we got lucky and found a few miracles at UMASS in Worcester.

Lesson: If something is wrong, or if pain continues, do what it takes to get help

Lesson: Doctors are human and make mistakes, so be your own doctor

Chapter 2

Three Months to Live

"He has three months to live." The medical staff doing the MRI was not encouraging and offered that assessment in an off-handed, clinical manner, not thinking about what those words meant to my family. My MRI showed that the great pain in my back came from an enormous tumor which had grown to touch all the key organs I needed to live ... heart, lungs, spine, liver, stomach... are there any others?

The tumor was also putting pressure on the nerves to my legs, causing spasms of pain so great I ground my teeth hard enough that fillings broke and fell out. For the last month or so I could not lie down or walk. I slept sitting up at a table while resting against a pile of pillows. My legs had swollen and I could not move them. I ground out my fillings from the pain, but could not lie back for my dentist to refill them.

Now, in the emergency room of UMASS Medical Center, something might be done. My wife, Mary Anne, had stayed by my side in the ambulance ride while my daughter Jean drove ahead to pick up my daughter Ruth. They all knew that the news was not going to be good, and so Jean and Ruth wanted to make sure that their mother was not alone when the news came.

The emergency room was undergoing renovations, so there were about 50 seats for about 75 people. Only one member of my family could be with me at any one time. The girls took turns while waiting for the MRI results.

The initial look at the MRI was not at all promising and an intern gave the off handed remark that "he has three months to live." I did not hear that prognosis because I was unconscious, knocked out by anesthetic and morphine due to the great pain. But my wife and daughters were there and awake at midnight. That news was devastating enough. But it only got worse.

We needed a miracle.

Chapter 3

A Tricky Operation

UMASS is a great teaching hospital, but they had no one in that night who could operate. My cancer tumor had grown so large it was shutting down the nerves coming out of my spine on the way to my legs. Every time I tried to walk or lie down the tumor would press against the nerves and cause a spasm of pain beyond anything I can describe. The tumor was shutting down the nerves ... slowly killing them ... and me.

But there was a tiny chance for a miracle ... and a miracle began to unfold. UMASS had just hired a new neurosurgeon, but he was not even due to start working at the hospital until the next week. This was early Wednesday morning and he was due to start on the following Monday. He was the only neurosurgeon available, and it was already past midnight when they called him. Luckily for me, when he heard what state I was in he did not hesitate and came in immediately.

But there was one little problem. He was not known by anyone at the hospital. He was so new he did not even have an ID badge and could not get into the hospital. Awakened at 2:00 AM, the Chief of Surgery authorized the doctor's entry and assured the hospital staff he was authorized to perform the surgery, even though he had never been in that operating room, and did not know any of the staff.

They say I came out of my drug induced stupor long enough to meet the surgeon, although I do not remember it at all. He told me I needed an operation immediately and I signed the consent form. The surgeon told my family to prepare for the worst. He said he had never seen such a massive tumor, and the MRI showed it had spread from my lower back to my upper back, an approximate distance of two feet!!!

"Even if he lives, he will most likely never walk again. He will be confined to a wheelchair." These were hard words to hear for the wife and family of a hiker, jogger and athletic man. My wife's instant response: "He may be paralyzed now, but he will walk. You do not know him. Just give him the tiniest of chances and he will walk." But that looked to be a near impossibility.

Our doctor devised a tricky procedure which he told my wife and daughters had to be done right away. It was going to be risky but hours might be all I had left to save my legs. Waiting until 8:00 AM for more staff might be too late to save what was left of the nerves.

How do you get a second opinion at two AM? My daughter Jean blurted out something like, "How do we know you are a good doctor? How do we get a second opinion?" Our doctor answered about the only way he could, "Jean, I am the only hope he has right now." And so he was.

He told me later that he was not able to reach the tumor directly since it was between my spine and my esophagus. It was impossible to access the tumor through the back because the backbone was in the way. The only way to reach it was through my side, a difficult procedure and a major operation. Rather, he tried to operate through the back just to relieve the pressure on the nerves enough to try to save them. He shaved some of the bone where the nerves exited the spine in order to increase the opening from the spine to help relieve the pressure. It was an operation that could not be termed normal or usual in any way, and thus there was no way to gauge if it could be successful.

At the same time he said he tried to get a sample of the tumor itself so the lab could determine the type of cancer to determine the best kind of treatment. Again, this was normally done from the side and usually could not be done from the back because the backbones are in the way. It was unlikely he could do all this, but if successful he would avoid a major second operation.

My wife and daughters stayed that night in the waiting room sleeping on a sofa and chairs. They consoled each other and wondered what the morning would bring.

After the surgery, our doctor gave a summary to Mary Anne, Ruth, and Jean. As he sat in a folding chair, the stark, unfinished waiting room seemed to be an appropriate background for his stark assessment. He reported that he felt he had relieved the pressure on the nerves, and that there was a slight chance I might walk again, although we would not know for days. Mary Anne said again, almost as a prayer, "Give him a slight chance and he will walk. You don't know Clint. Just give him an inch and he will find a way to walk again."

But at the end of the discussion the surgeon summarized by saying that he had never seen such a massive tumor, so, although he did not like to give results until all the tests were back, it did not look good. He advised them to prepare for the worst.

Chapter 4

Can You Move Your Toes?

I finally woke at about 7:00AM after being under for almost all of ten hours. I was overwhelmed by one sensation: the pain was gone. I had been living with increasingly severe pain for more than six months, a mystery to my doctors, and now it was finally gone. The relief was so great I was ready to get up and get going. But I realized something was not right. My legs were not working. I just assumed my legs just needed some time to wake up, and Mary Anne, Ruth, and Jean said nothing.

Shortly after I awoke, my team of doctors came to evaluate the results of their efforts. They first poked my feet with a needle, very gently, to see if I could feel anything. I could, which told them that some of the nerves were still in place, although they did not say anything at first.

Then they asked: "Can you move your legs?" No, I could not. I still did not appreciate just what was happening and the importance of the question. I had missed the last ten hours in a morphine-induced sleep when they figured out I likely could die, or probably be paralyzed and confined to a wheelchair for the rest of my life. "Can you move anything at all? Can you move your toes?"

I remember trying to get my toes to move and seeing that they would not. I would totally concentrate, and every muscle in my upper body would tense to its maximum, but still nothing would happen.

Only by repeating this maximum effort several times could I succeed in getting the tiniest of response in my toes. My pajamas and sheets were soaked in sweat from the effort.

As hard as I tried, I could move my right big toe maybe a half inch. I could move my left big toe too small an amount to measure, but we could all see it move. The doctors were ecstatic. I still did not understand what they could see and did not appreciate what it meant for weeks to come.

"If you can move your toes, then some of your nerves are not damaged. The good news is that some of the nerves are still in place all the way to your feet. Only time and therapy will determine how much of your nerve capability is still there and what will come back. We will have to wait and see."

Nerve damage? What will come back? I heard the words, but as important as they were I was too tired to understand them.

Oh, yes, by the way, you have a large cancer tumor in your back. Now this got my attention since I did not remember my morphine clouded conversations from the night before and had slept through the whole MRI procedure. They did not know the type of cancer yet. They were sure it was inoperable, but there was some hope it might be treated with chemotherapy. The lab results would be available in a few days. In the meantime they treated the tumor with a steroid, Prednisone, to shrink it while they tried to figure out how to treat it. "Don't worry, there are a lot of treatments, and we will find something."

Now I pride myself that my West Point training had left me able to handle just about any kind of bad news. But this was a lot to take in. A cancer tumor they might or might not be able to treat. Legs that were so paralyzed I could barely move my big toes and they were not sure how well I would ever walk again, if ever. My mind had yet to absorb this to understand the importance of what they were telling me. I had gone from morphine to Tylenol in less than twelve hours, but right now I was too tired to think. I had to sleep.

Lesson: Miracles can happen, so keep the faith

Chapter 5

Recovery Room Adventure

The next few days were spent in the recovery room in the hospital. The operation and the events of the past few months had left me more tired than I had ever been. I slept every night and most of each day.

For the first two days after the operation I was in the operating recovery intensive care unit, but not yet in the cancer ward. This location was a cause for nervousness because some of the patients were absolutely threatening. One in particular had been in a fight the night before and had temporary brain damage which caused him to swear constantly and threaten the staff and other patients until the nurses had to arrange for a police escort for him around the clock. This police protection was a good and needed step, but the bad part was that he was my roommate in a two man room and there were no other rooms available.

They moved him the second day, but Mary Anne stayed that first night. How my 5'2'' sweetheart thought she could protect me from a 6'2'' brain damaged whacko I do not know, but like it or not, she was better able to do so than I was.

On Friday the hospital physical therapist came by to evaluate my legs. She gave me ten exercises. I could do none of them. I could not lift my legs. I could not bend my ankles. I could not even wiggle my toes, except for minor movement of my big toes.

Her instructions were to do as many of the exercises as I could. I should try each exercise and have a family member assist with them as much as they could. For example, I should try to move my ankles back and forth, and since I cannot, have someone gently push them at the same time so the nerves can relearn what they are supposed to do. And repeat for your toes, and ankles, and knees, and so forth.

The therapist said she would come back again and drop in to advise me from time to time when she could, but weekends were difficult and she could not promise anything. Her advice was to exercise as much as I could if I ever hoped to get back the use of my legs. My situation was beginning to sink in, and tired as I was, I tried to repeat her exercises. But every set of exercises was so exhausting that after each set I had to sleep.

Saturday morning, the third day after my operation, my daughter Jean and her husband David visited. I was feeling a little better, after sleeping about 20 hours every day. We talked over what the therapist had said. Jean volunteered to assist with the exercises. I could barely bend my ankles, so she would let me start, then she would assist until we got them bent the full amount. We repeated this ten times. We figured out what we could do and adapted the therapist's instructions accordingly.

David set up a notebook with exercise charts so we could keep track; the first of what was to be dozens of notebooks. We repeated each of ten exercises ten times each for about 90 minutes worth of work. We repeated this in mid-afternoon. Sunday we repeated the exercise set, with Mary Anne taking over when Jean and David went home. This became our every day routine at least twice a day, and three times when I had the energy.

The several days in the hospital had made it clear how totally helpless I really was. I could not get out of bed. I could not move my legs without assistance. Nurses had to turn me over from time to time to change my sheets. I could not even get up to go to the bathroom but had to struggle with a bedpan. I could not get into a wheelchair by myself. I still was so tired I slept most of the time, and so it took a lot of time to settle into my brain how helpless I had become.

A few days after the operation, a friend dropped by with flowers. Friends from home sent a nice bouquet of flowers, and now Rita called at 6:00 PM to ask if it was OK if she dropped them by. I was tired, and Mary Anne and I had decided to limit visitors because that is always an additional tiring event, but for Rita we made an exception. She is one of our older friends. I thought I could stay up for the half hour or so her trip would take.

She should have been there by 7:00 PM, so by 8:00 PM we started to worry. I was dozing on and off when at 9:30, she called from the lobby. She had been lost, but she'd made it. My first thought was that I was too tired to see anyone, but I agreed for her to come to the room, and I was glad I did. I was not sure why at the time, but the kind thoughts from those still at home helped enormously to keep up my spirits.

The next day I agreed to let my five-year-old granddaughter and seven-year-old grandson visit. I had not wanted them to see me in my helpless state, but my grandson had tried to sneak into the car so he could come to the hospital to see me. It made me realize how much they were worried about me and needed to see me. These two kids began coming to see me three or four times a week, and it really was a morale booster every time I saw them.

I realize now, some years later, how close I was to these two grandkids. They were born in Seattle, the opposite side of the continent from Massachusetts. But I had been able to see them nearly every month for the three years before they moved back. This was because I had a subcontractor near Seattle for which I was responsible, so I had to take the long plane ride to Seattle each month.

Naturally, I stopped by to see my grandkids and I stayed with them each time. On reflection, since Mary Anne and I were the only family members that were able to come to see them regularly, we grew to be very close. And now they felt they wanted to see me, to help any way they could. And they did a lot to help.

Lesson: Visit your friends or family when they are in the hospital

Chapter 6

Hope from the Lab

Now that I was in the hospital and had had the operation, we knew what was wrong. I waited each day for word from the lab about the results of the testing of the sample that my doctor had been able to take. After five days my cancer doctor was able to tell us. He is a no nonsense doctor who had done significant research toward a cancer cure before joining the UMASS medical Oncology group for cancer treatments.

"We have some very good news. The surgeon was able to get a sufficient sample of the tumor for the lab to identify it. The lab confirms that it is a non-Hodgkin's lymphoma, the kind that we can treat effectively with chemotherapy." He began chemotherapy with Retuxibam, cyclophosphimide, vincristine, and prednisone, a combination that is particularly effective against this kind of cancer.

There are risks, of course. One can be intolerant of the drug, in which case other drugs would have to be tried. A relatively "minor" issue was that each treatment would cost about $20,000, and I would need four sets each month for four months then repeated as necessary for about a year. I was not so tired that I could not add up to over a half million dollars. This was a rude awakening to the world of big medicine finance.

Looking back, my attending nurse/guardian angel Mary Anne asked so many questions and did so much internet research that she became somewhat of an expert in insurance matters. In particular, she became our insurance system advocate/interface. It soon became clear that for every one of the several thousand hours of exercises I did in rehab, she spent an equal number of hours trying to straighten out the insurance billings and trying to arrange for the appropriate care.

At one point on one visit to a specialist's office the doctor complimented her on her knowledge of the insurance laws and procedures asked her if she could come to work as part of his office staff to handle insurance claims. Tempting, but her days were full.

Before the first chemotherapy I had to have a CAT scan. The machine for this is a large x-ray that takes hundreds of x-ray images of your body and produces images that look like individual slices of your body. The procedure was not too bad, but there was only one machine at UMASS at the time, and it was needed by a lot of people. So they wheeled me down in my bed and I slept in the hall for some time until it was my turn.

The next day came time for the first dose of chemotherapy. I knew this was the big test. If I could tolerate this drug I would have a good chance of beating the cancer. If not, things would get more difficult. In the cancer center I could see about twenty other patients getting the intravenous tubes dripping their cancer drugs into their veins. Some were having reactions … red faces, rashes; one had to stop the doses because of the reaction.

I was set for a six hour session. Everything was fine. I did two crossword puzzles, and then fell asleep. Mary Anne woke me for lunch

… she had sandwiches from the hospital cafeteria. I was lucky, I had no reaction whatsoever. Another hurdle passed.

Lesson: Talk to everyone and learn everything you can to find the best options

Chapter 7

A Ticket to Rehab

At day four after my operation, the hospital had space to move me to the cancer ward, and it was a lot quieter than the intensive care unit. The hospital could keep me only until the end of a week and had to move me to a rehab hospital for therapy. This raised two issues. The first was the insurance ... if you do not have insurance, no one will take you. Wow. But thankfully we have good insurance.

The second thing was the prospect of recovery. If you are fully paralyzed and not making recovery progress, you do not go to a rehab as it is a waste of time ... I am not too sure where you do go. Luckily I never had to find out.

Mary Anne and I had been working my legs diligently two to three times a day for the past week and I had made progress. I could move my toes and ankles ... not fully, but clearly. In fact, it was clear I could move most of my leg muscles, although most of them just a tiny bit. Most of my muscles had become weak from inaction for the several weeks prior to the operation. But they were moving which meant that most of the nerves were still functioning. This was great news that I appreciated more over the next six months.

While I slept, about 20 hours a day, Mary Anne stayed busy. She talked to anyone who would listen and asked as many questions as she could. She learned the ropes in a few days and figured out what the next steps might be. In particular she learned about the rehab options.

Two therapists came in to evaluate me on Thursday, one week after I entered the hospital. This was a key event because Mary Anne had learned we wanted to go to Fairlawn, the best rehab hospital in the area, but could only do so if they thought they could help me progress (and if our insurance was OK, which it was). The therapists tried each of the ten exercises. I could start them all, and do some of them all. Not fully, but enough that it was clear I just needed a lot of rehab work, which they are good at.

One of the therapists said, "This is not the man they wrote about on the initial evaluation. He is not fully paralyzed at all." I knew I had made progress. We were going to Fairlawn.

I still did not know the road ahead, and thought I would be up and about in a couple of weeks. Little did I know I had barely begun the process.

Lesson: Learn as much as you can about the best places to get the treatment

Chapter 8

A Wheelchair Brings Freedom

The next big challenge at the hospital was learning how to get into a wheelchair after being bed ridden for a week, and after having been unable to walk for three weeks prior to going to the hospital. I had always had a bad feeling about wheelchairs since they are a sign of paralysis and of lost mobility. But now I looked forward to the wheelchair as my ticket to freedom from lying in bed all day.

But in my state, getting into and out of a wheelchair was a project. I needed two nurses' aides or nurses to help me. The procedure was very inconvenient. First I had to call the nurse and then wait for her to find an aide. Second we had to park the wheelchair next to the bed and lock the wheels. Then the nurse had to use a three foot wooden "transfer board" to slide me from the bed into the chair. Then they had to essentially lift me onto the transfer board and then slide me over to the wheel chair, being careful to keep me from falling onto the floor.

This procedure was not something Mary Anne and I could do by ourselves for several more weeks. It was severely limiting to have to call for two attendants to get into or out of the chair since they were usually busy, but it was better than staying in bed.

I was fortunate in one thing. My upper body is in good shape and my arms remained strong enough to lift my legs and to drag my body around. My years of exercising and lifting weights really paid dividends here.

One problem we began to run into was something you would never think of. When you lie in bed, it is really helpful to raise your head for a while which a hospital bed can do. Each bed has a control panel to tilt you upward, which helps when you are eating, or reading, or doing anything but sleeping.

The difficulty with tilting is that you slide down the slope of a tilted bed; a little known inconvenience that healthy people never become aware of. But just try pulling yourself back up. You need to call for two nurses who drag you back up to the right spot. I was lucky and learned I had the upper body strength to do this on my own almost from the first day.

I was happy to be alive, and happier to be semi-mobile. But the difficulties of getting into and out of a wheel chair gave me a strong incentive to increase my muscle strength to gain more independence.

Lesson: Stay in the best health you can to meet the inevitable medical challenges ahead

Chapter 9

Rehab Challenges

One week after entering UMASS Medical Center I was on my way to Fairlawn Rehab Hospital. I was still nearly entirely confined to a bed, so this was an ambulance ride with me strapped into a bed. Two attendants arrived in my hospital room, strapped me in, and then wheeled me in my bed into the ambulance.

Fairlawn once was a beautiful old mansion with acres of lawns. It was turned into a hospital about fifty years ago, but then converted again to a rehabilitation hospital in 1985. The hospital itself is well kept, and the property is pleasant. It is a quiet, well run place, with great facilities for the exercises I would need.

My neighbor, Charlene, is a manager for visiting nurses for an insurance company. She knows all the hospitals in Massachusetts. She told us to get to Fairlawn no matter what. We requested it, worked on our exercises to get ready, and made sure our insurance was adequate, so Fairlawn was where we were able to end up.

I expected to be there four weeks, until the end of August, and home by Labor Day weekend. One month should do it, and I had things to do. Our initial stay at Fairlawn was set for four weeks as this was a typical recovery time for a stroke victim or an accident victim. I could live with that. Hey, I had no pain and was beginning to use a wheelchair; how much longer could this take? Boy was I in for a shock.

Fairlawn assigned Heather as the senior physical therapist in charge of my progress. Heather, we found out, was the one they assigned to the hardest challenges. She was responsible for understanding my condition, then devising the appropriate treatment, which consisted of exercises to strengthen various muscle groups. I was ready. I had always stayed fit my whole life by jogging, playing sports of various kinds, walking several miles every morning, and lifting weights. Give me the exercises and I will do them.

Fairlawn also assigns one occupational therapist to teach the patient the best way to deal with their limitations. Again, I was assigned to the guy who gets the most challenging cases, a huge man who could carry me if necessary. Dan had to be 6' 3" and weigh 300 plus pounds, and when he said we were to do something, there was no argument.

We met Dan first thing in the morning. He asked what we wanted to do first, as if I had a clue. Mary Anne did. "He needs a shower." I remember only how difficult this was. Dan could slide me into the wheelchair by himself, but I had to do the shower. I could not stand or move my legs. There are benches in the special showers. But each step of the shower was an ordeal.

Make sure you turn on the water before you get out of the wheelchair and onto the bench so you do not accidentally burn yourself if it is too hot (you cannot get out of the way). Drag your legs using your arms, one leg at a time. Toweling off after the shower was another learning experience that required eight towels since there is no way to stand, and the towels kept getting soaked. It seemed like hours, but I was finally done. I needed a nap.

But there was no time for a nap. Dan told me to get on my gym shorts and sneakers for exercise therapy. I had not dressed myself for several weeks now, but Dan insisted I learn to do so without help. If you want a real exercise in frustration, try dressing while lying in bed without moving your legs except by pulling on your legs one at a time with your arms. I think it would classify as a highly aerobic exercise routine, and at the end of it I was sweating so much I needed another shower. Just try putting on one sock while lying down and not moving your legs. But I learned to do it, better and better each day. And Mary Anne had to just sit there and watch in case Dan was spying on us to find out if she was helping.

Learning to get into a wheelchair was a big improvement. It took me about a week to learn to do it by myself to a level the nurses agreed that I could do so unattended. I could sit up OK, and then use my arms to pull myself near to the wheelchair. We learned to leave it locked near to the bed so I could reach it and drag it into position. Then I would place the transfer board from bed to chair and use my arms to pull myself over. As tricky as this was, I was very careful to avoid falling and luckily never did.

Transferring by myself meant that I could now get out of bed by myself when I wanted to and begin to wheel myself around the immediate area. I still had to be careful, since I could not really recover from an unlikely fall. But just getting up and out without having to call for nurses made me feel like I would eventually get out of there.

I also had an assigned nurse at a station near to my room to administer pills and to help with things like bed pans, water, meals, and questions. I was more fortunate than anyone else since Mary Anne stayed with me most of the time and made sure I was able to get the things I needed.

Lesson: Recovery will not be easy; work hard at it, especially when no one is looking

Chapter 10

Exercise: the Key to Recovery

My first meeting with Heather was an evaluation of my legs. In an hour she tried many exercises, most of which I could not do at all. I could hear what she wanted me to do, and I could try, but my legs were not responding. I could feel some muscles contract, but there was not enough strength to move them.

To give you some idea of where I was, I was assigned once a day to an exercise group of about ten wheel chair bound patients. These were accident victims, or stroke survivors, or people recovering from operations.

The exercises we were given for the legs consisted of sitting in the wheelchair, then moving one foot forward about twelve inches, moving it backward, moving it left, moving it right. These are so simple they are not even exercises except in name only. But I could not do any. The harder ones were raising your left leg, raising your right leg, crossing your legs left, crossing your legs right. These were things I could not even try.

In that first evaluation meeting with Heather, she asked what my goals were. I told her I intended to walk out of there. Heather did not say anything. She just looked at me and changed the subject. I assumed she was thinking I was at least saying the right thing. What she thankfully did not tell me is that they had never had a patient re-learn to walk again once the patient had forgotten how to walk.

Heather and Dan worked together on the exercises. It soon became clear to them that they could not use a standard set of exercises. My brain had forgotten how to use the muscles in my legs to do any activities. I could move the muscles one at a time, so we could tell that many of them were working OK. Also, I had a lot of feeling in all parts of my legs. The difficulty is that my brain had forgotten how to use the muscles together to do things like stand or walk. Heather and Dan began to realize they had to invent their own exercises and their own routines.

The normal rehab exercises for stroke victims or accident victims always included walking with a walker, a four legged device that allows the patient to walk while holding on to the walker for stability. In the first few days I found I could hold myself upward on the walker by using my arm strength to carry nearly my full weight, but my legs were unable to hold me upward, and unable to move in any coordinated manner.

After a few attempts at this, Heather and Dan decided to put aside the walker and just work on strengthening the leg muscles one by one. They devised a longer routine of exercises that I did twice a day under supervision, and suggested more exercises to do by myself when I could in the evening when we were alone.

Mary Anne was there every day watching and learning the exercises. Each day we had one set in the morning and another in the afternoon under the supervision of one of the many therapists, depending on their schedules. Mary Anne and I got into the routine of adding a third set by ourselves in the evenings when the therapists had left for the day. As hard as this was, the therapists all made it clear that the more I could work out, the better. The effort left me tired every night, so I slept well.

By the third week, it was clear that I was getting back some of the strength in my muscles. The exercise routines were getting easier to do, and Heather was adding heavier and heavier exercises. Dan showed me how to use the exercise bikes with tension controls, something we could do every evening. Progress was steady, but slow. I still did not understand the enormous hurdle I was facing, the one they were beginning to see, and I would not understand well for months to come.

Lesson: When a therapist gives you exercises to do, do them as often as you can

Chapter 11

The Cancer: Progress

I almost forgot about the cancer. I was so concentrating on the exercises and the rehab every day that the thought of the cancer did not enter my consciousness very often. And when it did, I never had concern about it. There was nothing I could do, so why waste time thinking about it. I was struggling to regain the use of my legs.

Every other week one day was cancer treatment day. Mary Anne found out that I could ride in a wheelchair. It is more convenient in a lot of ways and more flexible than being strapped in a bed since the wheelchair vans are more available. A significant factor was the cost, and since we were still not entirely sure who would cover what costs, we wanted to use the wheelchair vans since the ambulance rides are almost ten times as expensive as wheelchair van rides.

First thing in the morning the wheelchair van would come by and wheel me in for a ride to the cancer ward at UMASS for chemotherapy. This day always included a lengthy set of lab tests for seemingly everything they could imagine.

Once in the cancer ward, they moved me into a recliner chair and began the six plus hours of intravenous drippings. The doctor and nurses got to know us well over the next two years. They saw me start out by being wheeled in for treatments. They got snapshots of my progress every two weeks at the start, then moving to three weeks, and eventually to once every three months.

The chemotherapy treatments were enormously costly at about $20,000 every other week. We were getting the bills, but still were not sure of the reimbursement rules. I was spending three to four hours in rehab every day, while Mary Anne spent three to four hours trying to find out if we would survive financially.

Cancer treatments are nothing you can do anything about. If the treatments work, you are lucky and you will live a good life. If they cannot find the right treatment for the type cancer you have, or if it is untreatable, there is not a lot you can do. The best thing to do is to trust your doctors and ask everyone who might have useful information. There are lots of new treatments coming along every year, so hang on and hope you get a little lucky.

Lesson: Only worry about what you can control

Lesson: Concentrate on improving your health and leave the cancer to your doctors

Chapter 12

Coffee at 6:15 AM Every Day

At Fairlawn, Mary Anne and I settled into a routine. I had one advantage over every other patient at Fairlawn. Mary Anne was able to come in every morning at 6:15 with a Dunkin' Donuts coffee and a newspaper. This was a tremendous boost to our joint morale—to be together every day. It gave me a great start to a heavy workday.

The day nurses and staff came on at 7:00 AM. They had to first find out any changes that might have occurred with their patients, then make sure the meds were done, then clean and dress the patients, and finally make sure they had breakfast delivered to the rooms by 8:00 AM.

In contrast, Mary Anne would help me get up and help me to get dressed by 7:00 each morning. She gave me minimal help since Dan insisted I dress on my own, but she helped where she felt it was okay. Then we would get me into my wheelchair and out of my room before the day nurses had arrived for the day.

This early start was a great help. We would move into the open common area with views of the Fairlawn grounds and flowers. The nurses' aides learned to deliver my breakfast tray out there instead of in my room. Coffee, breakfast, paper, and Mary Anne's visit were a great way to start the day, especially out of bed and in a pleasant setting.

Of course, the nurses never forgot where I was when it came to my meds. The chemotherapy side effects included a spike in my blood-sugar levels to borderline diabetes. Every morning they would take my blood sugar, and if it was too high, I would get an insulin shot. If it was low enough, they would give me a pill instead. But they never forgot.

My early start to the day came about by an extraordinary coincidence—Fairlawn rehab hospital was located less than two miles from my daughter's house. So Mary Anne was able to live there while I was going through rehab. My son-in-law got up every day at 5:30 am to get to work by 6:30, so he woke Mary Anne and dropped her off on his way to work.

Mary Anne got in at 6:15 each day and stayed until 6:30 in the evening—twelve hours almost every day. The day-shift nurses came in after she did and left before she did. Many of the staff thought she worked there. She bought three meals a day at the cafeteria, and they knew her so well they assumed she worked there and automatically gave her the employee discount.

Mary Anne often spent much of the day chatting with the other patients and their visitors while I was exercising or napping. It got to the point that she was comforting some of the wives of some of the patients and offering hard-won advice to others. She became good friends with many of the nurses and aides as well as the accounting staff and management. She got to know them so well that on the day we finally left to go home, they bought her a beautiful spread of flowers to say good-bye.

From the first we limited our visitors. A lot of people asked to come, but we both knew that visits would be tiring, and I needed every ounce of energy I had to do the exercises. So we only permitted family and our neighbor Charlene to visit. That August my two grandkids and daughter came over most days for an hour or two. We usually played cards, hearts or crazy eights or old maid, until they had to go home. We also watched the first few innings of the Red Sox games. As luck would have it, the Red Sox had a phenomenal 2004 season to win the World Series, so this made for a great diversion.

I received over 150 get-well cards, a few each day. Each one was appreciated. But one Hallmark card, from Pat and Bob Green, gave me such inspiration that I read it to begin each day, and two or three times more after that, daily. It said:

I'm strong enough to rise above most any troubled time.

Today may be a mountain, but I was born to climb.

Funny how things work out, but a year later, when Bob had cancer, I bought the exact same card and sent it along with a note of thanks. A few months later I had occasion to stop by their house and noticed the card still tacked above his desk. That's where I keep mine, years later.

After being at Fairlawn for three weeks, I passed a test that showed I could work the wheelchair by myself well enough to have access to all hospital floors as well as the hospital grounds, something most patients there are not able to do. There is a lovely gazebo on the lawn far enough away that most patients could not get there. Mary Anne and I could, and we spent many pleasant hours there.

Lesson: Plan things to keep busy and to keep up your spirits.

Chapter 13

Mary Anne's Cancer

My cancer brought back memories of Mary Anne's cancer from ten years earlier. Her breast cancer had been an emotional trauma for us both. We feared the worst, which seems to be the natural tendency for everyone with cancer. Even though the survival rate for breast cancer was about 80% at the time, the fear of the worst outcome consumed our thinking. How could it not?

We have been a couple for a long time, since we were High School sweethearts so many years ago. We are soul mates: we think alike, share the same goals, enjoy the same things, and enjoy chatting about everything. Fearing the worst possible cancer outcome was not pleasant.

Never mind that we had the best of doctors. Never mind that they assured us that we had discovered the cancer early and that it was small and non-aggressive, and the chances of survival were excellent. We had heard all the stories of what breast cancer can do, and had even watched one friend battle it unsuccessfully, and so there was little that could set our minds at ease.

Our doctor was tops. Once we discovered the lump, she scheduled a biopsy within two days. But this brought only more questions. It showed that the lump was cancer all right and not something more benign. But now something more was needed.

Our emotions moved higher, from concern to fear, and at times sheer terror. Not knowing what would happen and having to wait was the hard part. We had always worked together to understand our problems and to deal with them, but this was out of our control.

The next step was another operation, a lumpectomy to remove the cancer. Since it was a small lump, about one centimeter, that was what the lumpectomy was designed to deal with. We had to wait and worry for three weeks, but with a good doctor we felt as comfortable as we could.

So what do you do while waiting? We gradually learned to stay busy and to live our lives as normally as we could. While the concerns were always there, we were able to put them out of our conscience most of the time. Still, the worries surfaced.

Then came some bad news. The lumpectomy confirmed the cancer, but the margins around the cancer were not large enough to give certainty that everything had been removed. The doctors suggested that another lumpectomy might be enough (about 65% certainty) but the only sure way to get rid of the cancer was a mastectomy to remove the entire breast. That decision was easy, and we scheduled the mastectomy.

Again, the waiting was the worst of it. Another three weeks of worry. But by now we had learned to deal with it as best as could be expected. We had learned to accept the fact that there was little we could do except to trust our doctors. Given that, we had learned to add as much as we could to our lives so that we had little time to think about the possible bad outcomes. We learned how to live without letting the cancer control our life.

When Mary Anne woke from the final operation, we both had a sense of relief. There was a lot of watching and waiting for several more years, but no need for radiation or chemo since there was no evidence that the cancer had spread. While this was a good outcome, the memories of this episode were still clear ten years later.

With my cancer, the story was much different. The medicines used to treat it were just a year or so past experimental, and so were still being monitored for side effects and for effectiveness. In my case they worked, and the tumor is no longer in evidence at all. But these drugs were not available ten years earlier at the time of Mary Anne's cancer.

In talking with our doctors we learned that many, many new drugs and treatments are on the way. My doctor told me that if this drug did not work, there were seven more under test. He was confident that one would be found.

This lesson is more difficult to phrase correctly. Some cancers are found too late to be treated effectively. But for most cancers, particularly those found in the early stages, help is possible. And for many others, help is coming.

Lesson: Do not let your fears control your life since the chances of survival can be good and may be improving.

Chapter 14

Reality: Will I Ever Walk Again?

Things were not going well after four weeks. I should have been getting ready to go home, but I was not ready. My muscles were getting stronger, but something was wrong. I was not learning to walk.

Heather and Dan tried everything they could think of. For several days we got down on the mats and tried crawling, which I found did help. Hey, that is the first step babies do when learning to walk, so why not? One little problem with this was that once I was on the mats on the floor is was difficult to get up since I could not use my legs, but that turned out to be minor. Dan just picked me up.

Day by day there were many signs that things were not progressing well with my legs. I could move one leg forward at a time, but that was done by cheating in a sense. I would twist my body to move one leg forward, while balancing myself on the walker.

On one occasion I fell over with my walker while moving down the hall. The nurses and therapists all came running to help. But there was not any good way to put a spin on it. I did not have the balance to stand up, and I did not have the wherewithal to control my legs.

When I really knew I was in trouble was the time I fell while playing Scrabble. We had a series of exercise classes with six of us who were just learning to stand again. Standing normally is an activity that people do without thinking. I could stand with great difficulty, but only with total concentration.

Our exercise class consisted of standing for five minutes then resting for five, on and off for an hour. Since it was boring to just stand around we usually played a game like Yahtzee. The point was to learn to concentrate on something else and learn to stand automatically.

One day for a change we played Scrabble. I am a crossword addict and do at least one crossword puzzle a day, usually a NY Times Sunday variety. So I like Scrabble. The game was definitely not competitive, but at one point in the game I realized I could use all of my letters and show off a little. As I worked at it I forgot completely about my standing. All of a sudden my legs collapsed and me with them. Luckily the hospital policy required a therapist directly behind each patient, and also to fit each patient with a heavy-duty belt the therapist could grab if necessary. Dan was right behind me, and caught me just before my jaw hit the table.

This incident caused some re-assessment of my situation. It was clear that my muscles were getting stronger, but that I could not control them well enough to stand or to walk. The only conclusion from this was that strengthening my muscles was not enough. It was all good and useful effort, but it was becoming clear that my nerves had been damaged a lot more than was obvious at the start. You simply cannot learn to walk if key nerves are not there.

The doctors could not tell us with any certainty what this meant. They did not know exactly how long it would take for nerves to grow back, or even if they ever would. The only advice they could offer was to continue to exercise as much as I could because no matter how much the nerves did or did not grow back, stronger muscles would help me to walk as well as possible.

We learned from friends that nerve re-growth could take up to two years, and if they are not back by then, then it is likely they will never come back after that. I asked the doctors and one did some Internet research. She reported that nerve re-growth would happen at the rate of one to three millimeters a day. My nerve damage occurred at my mid back (the T-6 vertebrae) so getting re-growth to my knees would take about six months, and to my feet would take over a year ... if at all.

This was a setback that could be enormously unsettling if you let it. But Mary Anne and I looked at this as another hurdle. There were a lot of signs that I was going to walk again, perhaps with crutches or braces, but only continued hard work would get us as far as possible. We continued with our routine of one hour of exercises in the morning, one hour of exercises in the afternoon, and one extra hour after dinner when I had the energy.

At this time the therapists recommended another four weeks at Fairlawn. I had been away from home for six weeks and was anxious to get home, but I had a lot more to learn and a lot more work to do to improve. So, reluctantly, we agreed, what else could we do, four weeks it was.

Lesson: Never give up. Keep working toward your goals

Chapter 15

Fighting the Anger

It is not easy to keep despair from setting in. After my miracle operation I had come to expect continued and unending progress in my recovery. And I wanted it to happen quickly. All of the other patients came and left within a few weeks. But that was not happening for me.

From time to time Mary Anne and I would get into the discussion of "why me?" Why did the doctors not see for six months that the pain in my back might be something needing more that pain killers? As we learned about the medical diagnostics that are available, why did our doctors never prescribe a CAT scan or an MRI?

I had initially gone to my doctor for the pain in my back in the January before my July operation. He thought it might be a pulled muscle, or some age related condition similar to what he was experiencing himself and so he prescribed physical therapy.

By May I had a deep cough develop as the tumor impinged on my lungs. Their medical group did agree to see me on an emergency basis for the cough. The doctor gave me cough suppressants, but when I asked about the pain in my back she said that I would have to come back and make another appointment, although she gave me more pain killers.

In mid-June I visited my doctor and could not walk in to see him, but had to be wheel chaired in. The fact that I was wheeled in did not cause my primary care doctor for twenty years to think that this might be the cause for further tests. He knew I was a long time jogger, and that I had been walking every day until this pain developed. He did take x-rays, but they showed nothing, so he had no reasonable thought to look further.

In early July I called my primary care doctor and asked for help since the pain was so great that I could not walk to get into his office. I asked if he could send over someone to take a look and advise me on what to do. He told me they could not do that and that I should hire a van and schedule an appointment.

Believe me when I say the remembrance of these events can make you angry. Mary Anne and I spend hours calming each other down. Only the continued progress of my muscle strength and my growing independence in the wheelchair kept our anger from dominating our existence.

It made us angry when medical professionals, friends of ours, told us that prescription pain killers should not be renewed indefinitely without further tests. Usually the rule is three renewals maximum, and then something more should be done.

Then we heard that some medical groups may get rebates determined in part by not prescribing "too many" tests. Several members of the medical profession have volunteered this information to us from time to time as they hear our story.

Mary Anne used this knowledge to good effect at least once. We needed an extension for rehab, but rehab stays are expensive, so the insurance company was at first not at all convinced they should pay for it. The therapists had to justify the extension, but approval was no sure thing. Mary Anne talked to the insurance company many times.

She finally said something to the effect that "I also have heard that you may have not authorized an MRI early enough which is why he was in so much trouble." Whether from her insistence, or from the therapists' reports, or from the insurance company case manager just doing the right thing we will never know, but from then on there was no trouble with the insurance company covering all the expenses.

Like most normal people, my health was not a cause for concern for my entire life, and so I never gave it my full attention. Year after year my annual checkups were good and I seldom had problems. So I did not think much of it when my primary care doctor talked about my health for five minutes, and then about other things for fifteen. I should have focused better.

Talking through our anger helped both Mary Anne and me to keep it under control. The constant improvement in my condition kept us from getting too angry. The continued exhaustion from exercises kept me from losing any sleep over it. And every time my anger began to boil, I could always do another set of exercises.

It is natural to seek legal advice in a case like this. But one session with a good lawyer made it clear to us that suing would take a lot of time and even money and the chances for any redress were minimal.

The lawyer said that the doctor had taken many appropriate steps (x-rays) to find out what was wrong and our surgeon had volunteered that the x-rays showed nothing suspicious. There was no evidence the doctor had done anything wrong, and other doctors confirmed his course of action.

The rule seems to be: if no one dies or remains incapacitated, the likelihood of a significant settlement is small. Based on this assessment we elected to spend our time and emotional capital on rehab, with good results.

Another cause of anger might well be called the "Why me?" factor. Mary Anne and I always took care of our health. We never smoked, drank alcohol only occasionally, always walked and exercised and stuck to a healthy diet. How is it fair that each of us ended up with cancer? Particularly when so many people we knew paid little attention to their health, smoked habitually, or drank regularly and never had cancer.

I think my brother-in-law had the best answer for this question. He did cancer research for many years, helping to find cures, and his knowledge is impressive. My paraphrase of his advice goes something like this: getting cancer is mostly a random circumstance. It takes two problems in a cell to make it cancerous, and those problems can be caused by any number of things.

As he listed all of the things: cosmic rays, radiation, genetics, smoking, asbestos, chemicals, and many more, it became clear that much of normal living can inadvertently cause cancer to develop. The longer you live, the more likely you will get cancer of one type or another.

The best strategy to take in life seems to be to stay as healthy as you can. This means exercising daily. It means eating a healthy diet. It means avoiding or overdoing the things that harm your health like smoking and drinking alcohol. Doing these things will allow you to have the best chance to survive the cancer or any other adversity when it hits.

In my case, there is little doubt that the walking we did every day gave us the wherewithal to overcome the cancer and the months of paralysis it caused. The exercise was the key.

Lesson: Take your health seriously

Chapter 16

Home, But Still in a Wheelchair

After eight weeks of rehab I was finally released to go home. I still could not walk. But I learned to be mobile using my wheelchair. Rehab had taught me the techniques needed to get out of bed and into my wheelchair by myself. I could dress myself and wash myself. Basically, I could take care of myself without constant attention.

I had also learned to drag myself for short distances using a walker. I liked to think that this was walking, but looking back I know I was not walking at all. I was simply balancing myself on the walker and using my arm strength to carry my legs along. I could move my legs forward one at a time, so it even looked like a kind of walking, but I could not stand up well enough to take even one baby step.

I was barely mobile, but stairs were impossible. My son-in-law and my son had installed ramps into the house, so I could move into and out of the house with someone pushing me in the wheelchair. I could get into and out of bed, but I could not go upstairs to bed, and so I slept downstairs in our family room.

But at least I was home. Mary Anne and I began the struggle to re-acquire our life, by trying to work our way back into our activities. There was, however, one thing that consumed much of my time every day: exercises. Leaving the rehab hospital did not mean I could stop the three hours of exercises each day. I had learned, and I believed, that exercises were the only hope I had to recover as much as possible of my legs.

I had also understood that the nerve damage was a lot more than anyone could assess accurately, and that I could only work and hope. The work would bring back what could be recovered. The hope was that this would bring back more nerves than I had when I came home. This was the great unknown.

Rehab at the hospital continued twice a week in outpatient rehab. We continued at Fairlawn, even though this entailed a 45-minute drive each way. But they knew us, and they had a great facility, so there I stayed.

The outpatient therapists began a different regimen of exercises, designed to improve my leg coordination and to help me to relearn how to use my legs correctly. They also taught me exercises that I could do at home.

At home I began to walk every day as much as I could. Mary Anne set up a loop in the house from room to room. On my first full day I did nine loops with my walker, as much as I could, of forty feet in length. It took so much energy that I had to rest an hour in between each loop.

Looking back, I could have been very discouraged being able to walk only 40 feet at a time. This was particularly true since we were in the habit of walking each morning on a three mile walk, and adding a minimum of three miles of jogging each week. But 40 feet was better than nothing, and I had not been able to walk at all for about six months. Even if it could hardly be considered walking, when I had left home nine weeks earlier I could not get out of bed and walk even ten feet, so I looked at it as progress.

There was no time for despair. I felt I was in a race to recover what I could before it was lost permanently. As long as I could make progress I could stay positive and focused. I kept a daily log of activities and of progress.

Lesson: Exercise every day

Chapter 17

Learning to Walk Again

The first day home from rehab was September 21st. I was able to use my walker to drag myself around a 40 foot "course" nine times. After each trip around the course I needed to rest. This was the starting point, and I knew I would have to do this as many times as I could and for as many days as it took for me to re-learn to walk.

To keep track of my progress I kept a log of each trip around the course. Every day I tried to increase what I had done the day before. The first day I walked 360 feet. The second day I walked 480 feet. Friday I walked 570 feet, but my legs began to tighten up so I stopped.

Each day I also had to complete an exercise set developed by my therapists. These were designed to strengthen particular leg muscles. I did these sets twice a day, typically for about an hour each set.

The one thing I feared most was breaking a bone or tearing a muscle. I had played sports my whole life and so I well knew how much a broken bone could slow me down. I wanted to avoid sprained ankles and pulled muscles. But most of all I wanted to avoid falling such that something might break, like a leg bone or collar bone. The last thing I needed was a multi-week delay in rehab to wait for something to heal.

I felt that I could push as much as possible, but no more than my therapists recommended. This was not easy to determine, but I adopted the philosophy that I could work until I felt tired and then stop. Most accidents occur when you are over tired. Whether this was the right approach or not, I was able to avoid all broken bones, sprains, and pulled muscles for the duration.

Saturday I completed 630 feet, and Sunday another 810 feet. Monday I went outside via wheelchair for the first time to walk. I could walk on the blacktop driveway. But this extra effort to get outside and then inside was too tiring an effort, so I stayed in for weeks.

The wheelchair is an enormously inconvenient mode of travel. I can say first hand that it is a great emancipator for someone who would otherwise be confined to bed. But to get into a car is a real challenge. I could get into the wheelchair by myself using my arms to drag me around while balancing myself on my legs. Then I could wheel over to the ramps where I would make sure I eased the chair down the ramp slowly enough that I could stay under control.

Once at the car, I could pull myself into the passenger seat. Mary Anne would fold the chair and lift it into the back of the car. God bless her, but it weighed about 25 pounds, and she lifted it in and out at least twice a day. The wheel chair was a great emancipator, but using it every day is an incentive in itself to learn to walk.

Tuesday I completed 800 feet. Wednesday I completed 770 feet. I tried to increase my distance every day, but I was at my limit. Frustration never quite set in before I did 950 feet on Thursday.

October 1st I was able to walk a total of 1320 feet, a quarter of a mile. Saturday I did 1350. Sunday was 1800 feet, still on a walker, but moving right along. I also noticed that I could move all my weight to one leg and then to the other, a direct result of the exercise routines.

Monday the 4th I walked another 1800 feet, but noticed soreness in my right hip muscles. This was an alarm to me, so I took it a little easy the next day and did 500. Also, this was a therapy session at Fairlawn, so I was careful.

Wednesday I did 600 feet. Thursday, the soreness was gone and I did 800 feet. Friday was 1250, and I was still careful. Saturday, 1350 feet, but stiffness warned me to slow down. Sunday I did 600 feet. Monday I did 1000 feet. I was anxious to do more, but my fear of breaking or ripping something overcame my anxiousness.

Tuesday was 1100 feet. Wednesday I did another 600 feet and felt some soreness. Thursday was an outpatient therapy day, and 500 feet of walking. Friday was 1000 feet. Saturday: 800 feet plus some time on the stationary bike.

Saturday was almost the disaster I feared as I fell over trying to get into my wheelchair an easier way. I twisted my big toe and it swelled up some, but I was lucky and could keep on going. Sunday I slowed down to 200.

Monday the 18th: 1100 feet. This felt good since the whole week was spent trying to get back to 1000 feet, and also continuing with the exercises. The progress was slow, but by keeping the journal I could look back from time to time to be sure things were getting better and to measure my progress.

My therapists were watching. They were complimentary of my effort, and could even see some progress, but they were concerned that things were going more slowly than they would expect. It was a struggle, but we were beginning to see limits.

<u>Lesson: Keep a journal so you can see your progress</u>

Chapter 18

My Knees Do Not Work

Two months of struggle led to the conclusion that my knees were not working properly. As I walked on my walker I was conscious that my knees were hyper extending from time to time. I did not know why, and the therapists were not certain either. But their research and experience were leading them to see this as the limiting factor.

The best they could figure was that the nerves in my knees were not functioning correctly. It was most likely that they were damaged from the tumor. They would need to grow back, if they ever did. The nerves in the knees sense the knee position and automatically adjust to the balance position. Whether the nerves would grow back was clearly an uncertainty.

Further discussions with the therapists began to clarify where this might leave me. At worst I would be limited to walking with a walker to get the balance and stability I would need. I might be able to progress to braces to stabilize my knees and arm crutches to balance and to allow my arms to assist my walking. There was just no way to predict what would happen with the nerves and if they would grow back or if they did, then when that might happen.

The good news this week was that I learned to stand without holding on to anything at all. Standing without a walker was very big in my mind. Looking back at it, it was not a natural standing with anything like a natural balancing that the body is designed to do. But it was standing.

It turns out that my leg muscles had strengthened such that I could compensate for the lack of balance. I learned to crouch about six inches from vertical, and in this way my knees would not hyperextend and I could keep my balance. I could stand this way for about ten minutes, but that was the limit because it required so much muscle strength. But it was an encouraging development.

Our therapists recommended moving to arm crutches as a step forward from the walker. They brought out a pair of arm crutches for me to try. At their sight they seemed to symbolize the possibility of me never walking normally again. The crutches were bringing that thought into Mary Anne's consciousness, and she did not like it at all. Tears filled her eyes and ran down her cheeks. Still, arm crutches are a step forward from a wheel chair, and I learned how to use them in less than an hour since my arms were strong enough to easily carry my full weight.

Our therapists also began discussing the braces that I might need. The braces would all be designed to stabilize and supplement the knees. Mary Anne and I were not convinced just yet. I was still making some progress, and so I was not too interested in agreeing to braces at this time.

But the discussion of braces did help me to understand how my knees were working, or rather, not working quite properly. In particular, they were hyper extending, meaning they were bending partially backward. If this were to continue it could lead to problems in the knee that would degrade long-term mobility and utility, likely leading to arthritis.

As we talked, I decided to try sports knee braces. I had heard of two pro basketball players who had hyper extended their knees, and they could play with sports braces, so it was worth a try. Basketball knee braces are nylon stretch braces, and some have metal frames to keep the knees from hyper extending.

I found these braces helped enough that with care I could stand better. I began standing as much as I could, which still was only about 30 minutes a day. But how are you going to get better at standing except by standing?

The week of November 3rd, four months into rehab, I had a walking session with my original therapist, Heather. I can only say that it was like a reunion. She had seen me at my worst but had not seen me since September and now I was walking to some extent with arm crutches. While she was complimentary on my progress, she gently pointed out that I had a long way to go. Four months into my therapy and walking, and I still had a long way to go.

The good news for the week was that I could finally get upstairs in our house. I had been unable to get up stairs at all for six months. But with my strength coming back in my legs I was able to get up the stairs by going backward, sitting on a step, and lifting myself up one step at a time. I could finally sleep upstairs in my own bed.

Lesson: Use every tool available to speed your rehab and recovery

Chapter 19

Out of the Wheelchair: After Four Months

Thanksgiving was a great time that year. After four months of rehab I was making noticeable progress. Thanksgiving dinner was at my daughter Jean's house, which meant I would have to walk up stairs to get to dinner. I was able to walk up the stairs normally, in the sense of one step at a time. But I still needed to hang onto the railing with all of my strength and pull myself upward. Also, I had two men behind me to catch me if I were to fall.

Everyone else watched what was happening from the top of the stairs. When I reached the top of the stairs there were hugs and clapping and cheers all around.

A few days after Thanksgiving I decided to give up the wheelchair totally. I could walk with the arm crutches pretty well. I could also balance well enough on my arm crutches that this had become my primary means of walking. I decided that the progress was continuing well enough that we could end the struggle with the wheelchair every day.

With the arm crutches I began to walk outdoors on the road. The first time I tried this I learned the hard way that the road is not as level as the course we had set up in the house. It is much more difficult to balance on slight inclines than it is to walk on the level. So after my first few steps I lost my balance and fell onto the road.

This fall caused great consternation among our neighbors. One neighbor was driving past at just that moment and immediately stopped to help. I knew that Mary Anne and the neighbor wanted to lift me up, but Dan's comments kept her from doing so: I had to learn to do it by myself or I would always be dependent. It took a couple of minutes, but I figured out how to get up by myself. Luckily, no harm done, nothing broke, and no injuries occurred.

The Friday after Thanksgiving I set my personal best of 2300 feet of walking (half a mile) using the arm crutches, all outdoors and on the road, and my first time past 1500 feet in a day. Then on Saturday I set another personal best of 3700 feet, more than a half mile of walking, also outside on the road. After struggling for so long, being able to walk more than half a mile was cause for celebration. I could not say what allowed this but I had been unable to get past 1500 feet until this weekend. It must have been the turkey and pumpkin pie.

Sunday I got past 5700 feet. Monday I reached 6760 feet, well over a mile. I was exhausted at the end of the day, but on Tuesday went over 6280 feet. I was so sore and stiff that I had to take off two days straight from walking, although the exercises continued.

Little triumphs still came every few days. I found I could actually walk up and down stairs, finally, with something approaching normal motion. I still was only able to walk one step, then stop, then one step, then stop, all to ensure I had my full balance at all times. I also hung onto the railings tightly and used them for balance and also to help pull myself up with my arms. I was determined to avoid falling down stairs since in the rehab I had met several older patients who had fallen down stairs and needed months of rehab to get back to normal.

We still had the rehab twice a week. Our therapists were happy with my progress. The strength had improved a lot, as well as my stamina. But try as they might, they were not able to help me to walk normally. I was learning to compensate for my less than perfect walking by using my arms to help balance and to help move my body along. I had learned what I needed to begin to walk correctly, but I simply could not get my legs to hold me up and balance correctly.

By now it was five months. I was beginning to reluctantly question if I might be reaching a limit in walking. Being on crutches is so much better than needing a wheelchair that I was still happy from putting away the wheelchair. But I could see every day that I was not walking correctly, even with braces and crutches.

While I might be reaching the limits, I was determined to keep exercising and walking three hours a day. If there was any chance at all to get further and to walk normally, I would do all I could to get there.

Lesson: Never give up

Chapter 20

Support from Friends and Family

Friends and family provided a lot of encouragement and help during my rehab. Looking back, the most important thing that friends did was to invite us to our normal social events as if nothing had changed, and then to work to make it possible for me to attend.

One of our bridge groups asked us for our October bridge event even though I was in the wheelchair and could not maneuver inside a house. I was able to maneuver on a walker, although I still could not get up any steps. Several of the men were available to help me struggle up the few porch steps and into the house by lifting and pulling.

In this bridge group we change seats and tables every four deals, but things were set up such that I could sit once and not move and everyone else moved around me instead. When I needed a drink refill (diet soda) there were 20+ volunteers to help. Other than those small problems, everything worked out well.

Another bridge group meets each Monday night, rotating from house to house in turn. This was impossible for me to get to, so they offered to meet at my house every Monday night with each in turn bringing in the munchies, drinks, and dessert. One other slight concession: I was unable to serve the soft drinks, so we went to a help yourself arrangement. This lasted for about four months, until I could get up stairs and travel easily.

At a Christmas party with friends I was able to get into the host's house, but that was about all. I had progressed to arm crutches by then. But I still could not stand and chat for any time, so I had to sit. But that was just fine. Friends came and sat and chatted. I struggled with the crutches, but friends came and moved them as needed.

We were lucky. We were able to carry forward with most of our activities every day, while continuing with our three hours of rehab every day.

Lesson: Be there for friends and family in need

Chapter 21

Learning to Stand

I learned how to walk out of doors that winter in spite of the snow, cold and ice. We found two strip malls in town with outdoor overhangs over the sidewalks connecting the stores. I could walk there with my arm crutches. There were patches of ice to avoid, and sometimes a little snow, but I never missed a day and I walked twice a day as often as I could.

Mary Anne would drive me to the mall and sometimes walk with me, and sometimes wait in the car. We measured the distance as one sixteenth of a mile, and I would walk back and forth as many times as I could. When I progressed to a mile, it would take about 25 minutes. Before long I was walking so much past so many stores that Mary Anne could do her grocery shopping and chores while I walked along outside. With this regimen the strength in my legs continued to increase.

I still could not stand normally. I found that the braces helped a lot by restricting my knees and preventing the hyper extension that might cause long term damage. In order to stand I had learned to compensate by flexing my knees slightly, standing in a semi-crouch. I could stand like this as long as I needed for all normal activity in life, but it was impossible to maintain this position for more than about ten minutes at a time without needing to sit down.

On Valentine's Day an unusual thing happened. I was standing up to eat breakfast as part of my exercises. But that day Mary Anne noticed that something was different. I was not in my semi-crouch, but was standing up straight for the first time in a year. I had been struggling with this for so long, and Mary Anne noticed it before I did.

For some reason things came together that day. Looking back at it, the strength in my legs had been coming back slowly but surely which probably explained it mainly. But also the nerves had likely regenerated from the area of the operation in my back, a distance of about 500 millimeters, which would have meant a 2.5 millimeter per day growth rate. This was within the range the doctors had given me. But whatever the reason might be, I could stand up normally.

Knees are complex things. While I am not an expert, I understand that there are nerves in the knees that help with automatic standing. The thigh muscles (front) are in balance with the hamstring muscles (back), and the nerves in the knees help to keep them in balance. I am not sure that I understand the exact process, but that was not necessary. What was important is that on Valentine's Day I could stand normally. While I did not appreciate this seemingly slight improvement at first, this was the breakthrough that eventually enabled me to walk and stand normally.

Lesson: some things just take time

Chapter 22

Beating Odds of 100,000 to 1

Learning to stand normally was the breakthrough I needed. It was a long time coming, but it was a huge improvement. Once I could stand normally I began to progress very rapidly with walking. At first I found I could take one baby step at a time, rebalance, and then take another. Amazingly, I did not need arm crutches to do this.

Within a few weeks I could do this with steps that were normal in length. I began to walk without the crutches at all, although I kept using a cane just in case I needed help balancing. I still did not want to risk falling and breaking something.

My therapists at Fairlawn were more than pleasantly surprised. They were quick to agree that I was learning to walk normally. Since I had overcome the standing hurdle, now the rehab lessons and exercises were aimed at overcoming the bad habits I had developed in the past six months while compensating for incorrect walking. My balance was good and I was walking correctly.

A few weeks after this improvement, Cindy, the lead therapist, took me on a test walking tour through the hospital and up and down some small hills outside. She said I had passed the test and that I did not need to come to rehab any longer. It was mid April, nine months after my operation and a full year after I had lost my mobility. But there was no doubt that I could walk normally.

On our last day, Cindy also said to us that in all their years as a rehab hospital they had NEVER had a patient re-learn to walk again once the patient had forgotten how. In her words, the chances against my walking normally again were a hundred thousand to one.

Those words explained a lot. In my six months at Fairlawn the therapists were all working hard to make me walk as well as I could, and they helped a lot. But none of them let on that my chances of walking normally were next to impossible.

Needless to say, we left Fairlawn on that last day feeling elated. It was April 12th, almost nine months from my operation, but I was walking again. I still had a lot of work to do to get my full stamina and strength back, but I thought nothing could stop me now. Winter had come and gone, and spring was here. Our outlook was optimistic.

Little did I know my troubles were not yet over.

Lesson: To learn to walk again, stand first, then take small steps one at a time

Chapter 23

Chemo Treatment Update

The chemo treatments continued every three weeks. The first treatment started right after the lab was able to identify the type of cancer that had struck me, within the first week of the operation. Each chemo treatment required a CAT scan first so the doctors could tell how the cancer treatment was progressing.

I never concentrated very much on the chemo treatments because our cancer doctor was encouraging and there was nothing we could do. The lab had determined that the cancer was a non-Hodgkin's lymphoma. He had determined that there was a drug that would attack that cancer type directly. There was not much else I could do, and so I trusted the doctor and concentrated totally on my health and my walking.

I had treatments at $20,000 each. Each one was administered at UMASS Medical Center and was an all-day session of intravenous drugs. After the first four treatments I could tell that there had been a major change in my body. In one two day period I lost eight pounds, mainly fluid. As an incurable optimist I just "knew" that the tumor had shrunk, and this turned out to be the case.

In December, after five months of treatment, our doctor decided we could stop the chemo since there was no longer any sign of any cancer anywhere. This was great news. This was the greatest Christmas present we could possibly have gotten. After all the struggle of the past year, we were glad that the end was seemingly in sight.

At the start of the chemo sessions our cancer doctor told us I might need chemo for a long time, as long as a year. We calculated that this would mean $350,000 in medical costs. It turned out that eight treatments were enough. It was a good thing that we had insurance that covered it all.

We were fortunate with our insurance. We had been in our own business for fifteen years and were always able to afford insurance, sufficient to cover major disasters such as cancer. I can only say that it was a worthwhile expense. As we watch the insurance debates, first in Massachusetts, and now nationally, insurance needs to be affordable for everyone.

Besides being fortunate with insurance, we were fortunate with our personal financial situation. We ran our own business, developing high technology discoveries I had made from time to time. I was semi-retired in that we had enough saved and invested that by living frugally we could do the things we wanted to do, and did not have to seek employment. Because of this fortunate circumstance, I could take the several months needed for a rehab stay in a hospital without worrying about a paycheck. Mary Anne could check the business emails and correspondence as necessary, but things moved along to our pace.

With cancer, the end is never in sight. We would need CAT scans and lab work every three months for years to come. This would continue to emphasize the importance of our insurance and our flexibility to meet our treatment needs.

Lesson: Make sure you have good insurance

Chapter 24

A Problem: Radiation Treatments

The radiation treatments almost killed me. The good news was that the chemo treatments were ending. The bad news was that radiation was about to start. The doctors all felt the same way. The chemo had worked very well, better than anyone could have hoped. But to be more certain that the cancer would never return they all recommended that I have radiation treatments.

The cancer effects mostly occurred at the middle of my back, the area of the T-6 vertebra. It was natural for the doctors to conclude that this should be where the radiation would best be applied. The theory was that there could well be microscopic cancer cells left over from the tumor, and they did not want to chance that some of them might begin to grow again.

The problem as I saw it was that this meant radiating me directly in the middle of my chest. The things that would be radiated were my heart, my lungs, my esophagus, and my spine. After all that I had been through I was not happy with this and did not look forward to it. I did ask for two second opinions, and all were the same: if your doctor says it will improve your chances, then you should do it. Think how you would feel if the cancer returned and you might have prevented it.

I had one of the best cancer groups in the world plan the radiation program, the Mass General Hospital extension at Emerson Hospital. They recommended twenty treatments; one a day for four weeks total.

Treatments began in late January. The first two weeks of treatments were relatively easy. The doctors said I could expect to be fatigued, but that did not happen at first. My walking rehab continued at a good pace. After two weeks of treatments my daughter-in-law gave birth to a granddaughter in the maternity ward in the same hospital, so we could stop up to visit after each treatment. This was something to look forward to at the end of a few radiation treatments.

However, after fifteen radiation treatments I did not like the way my body was reacting. I had pain in my esophagus, which was to be expected. My heart was getting irregular heartbeats and felt uncomfortable from time to time. Fluid was building up in my lungs, making breathing more difficult. The doctor explained that these symptoms were to be expected, along with tiredness and loss of energy. I found that walking was becoming more difficult, and after all the rehab I had been through, my walking became less and less every day. The last thing I wanted to do was to again lose the ability to walk.

After two more treatments, seventeen total, I told the doctor that I had had enough. My body was giving me a lot of signs that this was more than I could handle. The doctor listened, and then agreed that maybe seventeen treatments were sufficient.

Three weeks later we took a trip to Florida, a way to visit friends, but also to visit a company that was considering buying one of our products. The trip was a short one, just three days.

We landed back home on the day before St Patrick's Day. That night I began to feel very badly. I felt that my heart went into a very irregular beat I had never felt before in my life. I also was having great trouble breathing. For the first time in all my trials and troubles of the past year I felt a threat to my life and knew that something needed to be done right away. I called the doctor at 11:00 PM and he told me to head to the emergency room ASAP.

There they put me into the intensive care unit right away. My heart was in atria fibrillation, which we were soon calling A Fib for short, just like the doctors and nurses. A Fib is not good at all since it means that only half of the heart is working, and the blood in the other half is just sitting there. The IC doctors were concerned that if this kept up for long, a day or so, there was danger of blood clotting in the heart which could clog a healthy artery and lead to stroke or death. In addition I had fluid buildup in my lungs that was slowing down my oxygen intake such that I kept feeling like I could not breathe and was drowning.

The IC gave me blood-thinning drugs to prevent the clotting. They put me on oxygen to let me breathe better. Then in order to continuously monitor my heart they wired me up with so many electrodes I felt like Gulliver in the land of the Lilliputians. I had trouble moving.

All of this was bad enough, but the worst part is that I could no longer continue walking. I tried to keep walking, but the lack of oxygen and the heart arrhythmia limited me to a few baby steps at a time. I was disturbed a lot at this, but I recognized that I had to deal with this new threat and that it was serious.

I was in good care, thankfully, and so things progressed well enough, if a little too slowly for me. There was not a lot I could do, but by the end of two weeks my heart was back to normal, and the fluid had receded in my lungs. I was past the worst of this crisis after about a month. But it still was not over as I was to find out.

Lesson: Never get complacent, but just get ready for the next bad news

Chapter 25

The Aftermath: Diabetes

After my trip to intensive care things began to improve fast. I continued to exercise about an hour a day and walk about an hour a day. By summer my walking routine had returned to the 3 plus miles every morning that it had been before the pain had forced us to stop some eighteen months earlier.

By July, one year after the operation, I could take stock of what I had been through. There were still issues, but for the most part they were things that I could work around while I continued to improve. One item was that the nerve re-growth had not reached my feet, and so there continued to be partial loss of feeling in my toes. There were still strength and balance issues, which, again, were relatively minor things I could work to improve.

I continued to have good reports from my cancer doctor. Every three months I had a CAT scan and blood work and the other normal check-ups. There was not the slightest hint of anything out of normal, which was a great sign. There was no sign of the original tumor, which was remarkable, as normally there is a small tumor that remains in remission and requires observation forever. One doctor we had consulted was astonished that the tumor had completely disappeared and said he thought that was highly unusual.

But in the past year we had endured enough setbacks, large and small, that I remained cautions. I continued to work and exercise to improve my health as much as I could in order to get ready for the next problem.

One apparently permanent result of my cancer treatment was the onset of diabetes. There was no history of this in my family, but the drugs that were used in my treatment triggered the diabetes, something that is a common after effect. Because of this my doctor told me I needed to test for blood sugar levels twice each day, once in the morning and once at night. By monitoring the sugar level I could take appropriate action to keep the blood sugar within limits.

My diabetes level was probably best called borderline diabetes. While I was taking the steroid Prednisone my blood sugar levels were high, but when the Prednisone doses stopped, then my blood sugar was best described as "high normal."

There are two main ways to treat the diabetes. The first is with drugs. The second is with diet and exercise. I dislike taking any drugs because you never know what secondary problems they will cause for you while addressing the primary problem. So I agreed to take a minimal dosage of drugs and to work at diet and exercise while monitoring my blood sugar. This seemed like a good plan, and since I was already doing about two hours of exercise and walking I thought this would be simple. But it was not simple at all.

I began to research diabetes and its treatments in earnest. Here I turned to the Internet, and in particular to WebMD.com. This source directed me to as much information as I could use about the various medicines that would help, and the foods that I needed to be careful with. Even with this information I found that controlling my blood sugar turned out to be a daily struggle.

The best way to address diabetes is by watching the food intake. You do not need to go hungry, but you do need to cut out refined sugars, alcohol, and then cut way back on carbohydrates. I tried to do this at first by taking a "little by little" approach to give up only the worst of foods, while keeping most of what I liked.

This approach helped some, but the hard part was realizing that I really liked a lot of foods and drinks that could not be continued long term. For example, it was easy to give up most sugar-based foods like candy and sodas for sugarless candy and iced teas. I gave up refined flour based breads for whole wheat breads. It is not quite as easy to give up refined sugar based desserts like cookies and cake, but that too is do-able by substituting fruits. But portions of ice cream remained on the list at first.

Almost no one goes on a diet and stays on it for long. Just the thought of a diet conjures up visions of always being hungry such that most normal people react by binging and ultimately going back to their old eating habits. But it is workable to think of substituting some foods for other foods to eliminate sugars.

I worked at this substitution method with some seriousness, but I was still placing a higher priority on my walking and exercises. I did not yet appreciate how serious diabetes is. Diabetes is a long-term life threatening condition that has to be addressed seriously.

My diabetes was not so serious that I needed insulin. It was more a borderline case with some readings higher that I wanted, but with the long-term tests in the normal or near normal range. My doctor prescribed Glabouride pills at first, a drug that causes the body to produce more insulin and thus reduces the sugar in the body.

Glabouride was too strong for me. I tried taking it morning and night, but found I would actually drive my blood sugar so low it led to a low blood sugar reaction of major headaches and weakness. I cut it back to half a pill and that seemed to help, but the sugar low reaction problem did not go away.

For the second year after my operation I was more serious with cutting out some foods, and cutting back on others. But my sugar readings started to inch up little by little and this problem moved into the forefront.

Two years after my operation my doctor took a new look at my blood sugar and explained that my long term test showed I had moved into the diabetic range. He prescribed a less strong drug, Metphorin that would help me to avoid the stronger sugar-low reactions. Metphorin works to keep the body from producing sugar, compared to the Glabouride that produces more insulin.

This new drug and my own new priorities seemed to do the trick. The move into diabetes caused me to take my diet a lot more seriously. I went back over everything and found I had made a good start, but more could be done quite easily. So instead of reducing alcohol intake to occasional, I stopped it altogether. Instead of milk on cereal in the morning I stopped drinking milk since it has a surprisingly large amount of sugar. Instead of flavored coffee with half-and-half I began to drink it black. Desserts were only an occasional indulgence.

This new priority let me get back into the normal range in my tests within three months. This is good news, but this one will be with me forever.

Lesson: Take care of your health as a top priority

Chapter 26

A PET Scan: More Cancer

The next big shock came two and a half years after my operation. I had my first PET scan, which showed that I still had the cancer, although in a small tumor less than an inch in diameter. The good news is that it was not spreading or growing. The news of cancer still being there was unwelcome after two and a half years of improving health and rehab, particularly since I had been told it was gone.

This tumor did not appear to be a new tumor, but rather the identification as cancer of an existing anomaly by use of the PET scan's cancer identifying capabilities. The five CAT scans since my operation had allowed monitoring of five anomalies in various parts of my body. None had grown since my operation. But the CAT scan cannot identify anomalies as cancer, so my cancer doctor ordered a PET scan to provide improved cancer monitoring.

The good news is that the cancer was identified and located. It means it can be monitored better. If it shows signs of getting larger, it can be treated. It had not grown in two and a half years, so it likely is a slow growing type that will give plenty of notice, and will allow time for treatments.

While the news was unwelcome, it was not devastating by any means. I would even say it was not entirely unexpected news. One doctor we consulted had looked at the CAT scans and said he was surprised that the original tumor had disappeared from just the chemo treatments. He said that was quite unusual. But he was looking in the middle of the back, in the T-6 region, which was to be expected since that was where the nerve damage had occurred. This analysis stuck in my memory and I always wondered if the original tumor had just been shrunk.

This newly identified tumor was much lower, in the L-5 region, which is the lower back, and is a good eighteen inches away. It would be difficult to look at a CAT scan and connect the newly identified tumor with the original problems.

The PET scan is a better cancer identifier than a CAT scan. PET stands for positron emission tomography. Prior to the PET scan I receive an injection of radioactive sugar and sit still for about an hour while this sugar moves throughout my body. Research has found that cancer tumors absorb the radioactive sugar. The radioactivity then gives off positrons which are then mapped and show the location of cancer. This causes the tumor to appear "hot" on the PET scan.

I asked my doctor if the newly identified cancer might be the original tumor in a shrunken form. The short answer is that there is no way to tell. We are where we are and we can only go forward from here.

Lesson: Keep your health as good as possible to help yourself through the next crisis

Chapter 27

Three Great Years

My cancer and rehab was a three year struggle. But as I look back, I realize I lived through three great years. The best part is I lived to see three new grandkids to join my other three. Happiness is children, and I have been blessed.

I re-gained the use of my legs. Walking is vitally important to long term health. I beat one hundred thousand to one odds in re-learning normal walking after losing the use of my legs. That was the greatest struggle I have ever had to face.

I learned many great lessons that will help me from now into the future. Most important is the lesson of working every day to keep your health at as high a level as you can to be ready for the unexpected crisis that is certain to come your way. The best way to do this is to walk every day. The media is filled with articles on health, but the one thing that comes through above all others is that walking every day is the best exercise for the human body.

I learned to be my own doctor. It takes a bit of work, but anyone can find a lot of background information on WebMD.com to make themselves knowledgeable about their symptoms and conditions. Your doctor can help, but you need to know as much as you can.

I had always appreciated my family and friends. I know now that I needed their support and help in my time of need. They all came through, and for that I will always be greatly appreciative.

I am now back to walking three miles a day with Mary Anne. We do this first thing, before anything else at all. We have so many things happening that if we put off our walking until "later" it somehow never gets done.

I also firmly believe that I am in better shape now than I was before the cancer started. Part of that is the walking, but part of that is that I also do a set of exercises every day, inspired by my therapists.

As a final note, I would also like to think I inspired my doctor to some degree. He has lost 30 pounds, and he has started to walk every day. And so, hopefully, will you the reader start doing.

Lesson: Walk every day, at least 30 minutes

Appendix: Lessons Learned Chapter

Exercise every day   16

Keep a journal so you can see your progress   17

Use every tool available to speed your recovery   18

Never give up   19

Be there for friends and family in need   20

Some things just take time   21

To learn to walk again, stand first,

        then take small steps one at a time   22

Make sure you have good insurance   23

Never get complacent, but just get ready

        for the next bad news   24

Take care of your health as a top priority   25

Keep your health as good as possible

        to help yourself through the next crisis   26

Walk every day, at least 30 minutes   27

www.ingramcontent.com/pod-product-compliance
Lightning Source LLC
Chambersburg PA
CBHW031241280526
45784CB00004B/1669